MEDITERRANEAN DIET COOKBOOK FOR BEGINNERS 2024

Simple and Delicious Recipes for a Healthy Lifestyle

By

Hector Wiggins

Table of Contents

CHAPTER ONE

1 INTRODUCTION

In the enchanting realm of culinary exploration, where the symphony of flavors dances with the essence of well-being, we invite you to embark on a transformative journey through the pages of our "Mediterranean Diet Cookbook for Beginners 2024." Picture azure coastlines, sun-drenched landscapes, and the tantalizing aromas that waft through charming villages – this is the heart and soul of the Mediterranean diet.

As the sun dips below the horizon, casting its golden glow over olive groves and vineyards, we invite you to join us in embracing not just a diet but a lifestyle. Imagine sitting under a pergola, savoring the richness of a ripe tomato, the earthiness of olive oil, and the simplicity of a well-prepared meal.

This cookbook is your passport to this idyllic world, where the harmony of fresh, wholesome ingredients converges with the art of Mediterranean living.

Our journey begins with a narrative that unfolds the secrets of this time-honored diet – a tapestry woven with tales of longevity, vibrant health, and a celebration of the senses. Through these pages, we will demystify the Mediterranean diet, guiding you from the market to your kitchen, offering insights into the culinary traditions that have sustained generations.

Whether you're a novice in the kitchen or a seasoned home chef, this cookbook is a compass, guiding you through the diverse landscapes of Mediterranean cuisine.

From the sun-kissed orchards of Greece to the aromatic kitchens of Italy, each recipe tells a story – a story of connection, nourishment, and the joy that comes from savoring the simple pleasures of life.

So, with an apron in hand and a spirit of adventure in your heart, let the Mediterranean Diet Cookbook be your trusted companion. May these recipes not only fill your plate but also inspire a lifestyle that transcends the ordinary – a celebration of good food, good health, and the timeless joy of shared meals with loved ones. Welcome to a culinary journey that goes beyond the kitchen – welcome to the Mediterranean way of life.

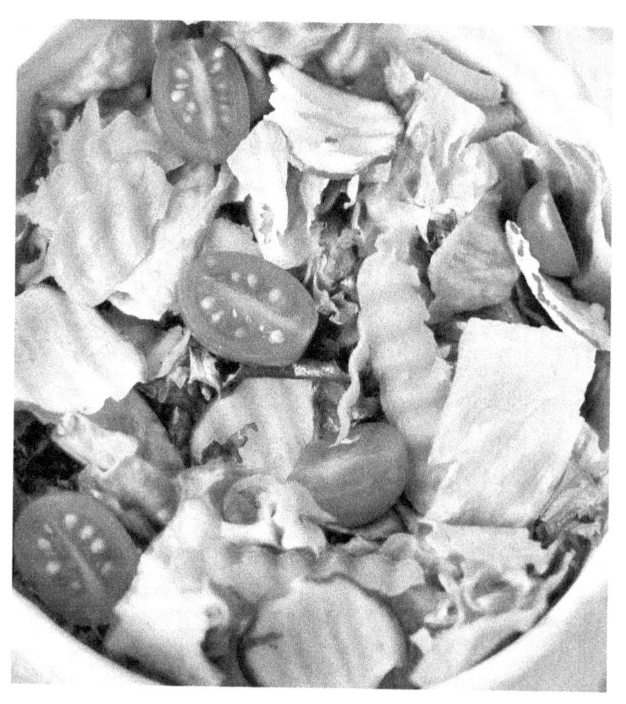

1.1 **Understanding the Mediterranean Diet**

Understanding the Mediterranean Diet goes beyond a mere list of foods; it encapsulates a holistic approach to nutrition and lifestyle inspired by the traditional dietary patterns of countries surrounding the Mediterranean Sea. This dietary philosophy has gained recognition for its numerous health benefits and its role in promoting longevity.

Foundation of Freshness: At the core of the Mediterranean Diet is an emphasis on fresh, whole foods. Fruits, vegetables, whole grains, nuts, and seeds form the foundation, providing essential vitamins, minerals, and fiber. These nutrient-dense choices contribute to overall well-being and support bodily functions.

Healthy Fats, the Mediterranean Way: Olive oil, a staple in this diet, is rich in monounsaturated fats, which have been linked to heart health. The diet also includes sources of omega-3 fatty acids, such as fatty fish, offering additional cardiovascular benefits.

Moderate Protein Intake: While there is a focus on plant-based proteins like legumes and nuts, the Mediterranean Diet includes moderate amounts of lean animal proteins, such as poultry and fish. This balance contributes to satiety and supports muscle health.

Savoring Seafood: Fish and seafood play a prominent role, offering not only protein but also valuable omega-3 fatty acids. These healthy fats are known for their anti-inflammatory properties, contributing to overall health.

The Power of Herbs and Spices: Beyond flavor, the Mediterranean Diet incorporates a rich array of herbs and spices, not only enhancing taste but also providing potential health benefits. These include antioxidant and anti-inflammatory properties.

Mindful Eating: The Mediterranean way of eating is characterized by a relaxed pace and an appreciation for the social aspect of meals. Taking time to savor and enjoy food fosters mindful eating, promoting a healthier relationship with food.

Moderate Wine Consumption: Red wine is a staple of this diet when it is taken in moderation. Because of its high antioxidant content, it is thought to have cardiovascular advantages. But moderation is essential because drinking too much alcohol might have negative consequences.

Physical Activity and Lifestyle: The Mediterranean Diet isn't just about food; it extends to lifestyle choices. Regular physical activity, shared meals with family and friends, and a focus on enjoying life contribute to the overall well-being associated with this diet.

Understanding the Mediterranean Diet, therefore, involves embracing not just a set of dietary guidelines but a way of life that promotes health, longevity, and the joy of savoring delicious, wholesome foods in good company.

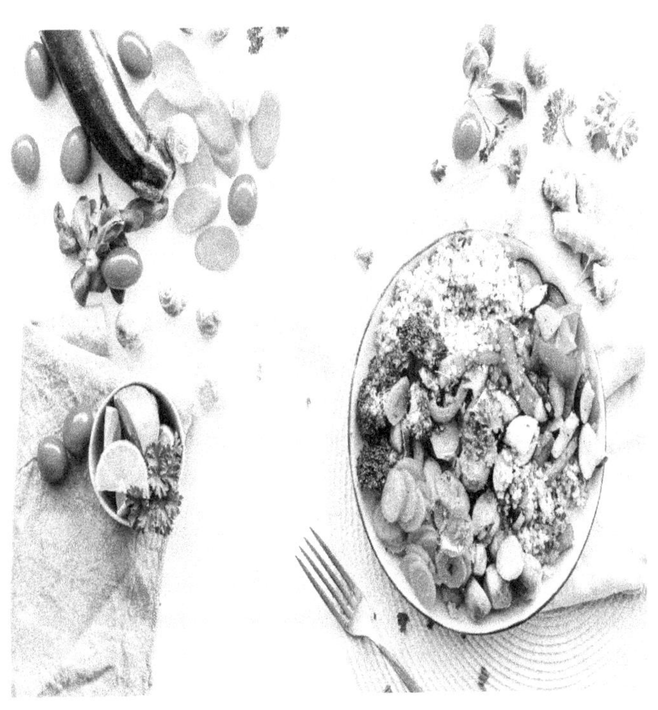

1.2 Health Benefits and Principles

The Health Benefits and Principles outlined in a Mediterranean Diet Cookbook form the cornerstone of a lifestyle that goes beyond just culinary preferences. These principles are rooted in the traditional dietary patterns of regions surrounding the Mediterranean Sea and have been associated with a plethora of health benefits:

Heart Health: The Mediterranean Diet is renowned for its positive impact on cardiovascular health. The inclusion of heart-healthy fats, particularly from olive oil and fatty fish, along with a focus on whole grains, contributes to lower risk factors for heart disease.

Rich in Antioxidants: Abundant in fruits, vegetables, nuts, and herbs, the diet is naturally rich in antioxidants. These compounds help combat oxidative stress and inflammation, playing a role in preventing chronic diseases and promoting overall well-being.

Weight Management: The Mediterranean Diet encourages a balanced and sustainable approach to weight management. The emphasis on whole, nutrient-dense foods and moderate portions supports healthy weight maintenance.

Improved Blood Sugar Control: With an emphasis on complex carbohydrates from whole grains, legumes, and vegetables, the Mediterranean Diet may help regulate blood sugar levels, reducing the risk of type 2 diabetes.

Brain Health: Omega-3 fatty acids from fish, as well as antioxidants from fruits and vegetables, are associated with cognitive benefits. The diet may contribute to a lower risk of cognitive decline and neurodegenerative diseases.

Inflammation Reduction: The combination of anti-inflammatory foods, such as olive oil and fatty fish, helps mitigate chronic inflammation, a factor linked to various diseases, including arthritis and certain cancers.

Digestive Health: High-fiber foods like fruits, vegetables, and whole grains promote a healthy digestive system. Additionally, fermented dairy products, common in the Mediterranean Diet, can contribute to a balanced gut microbiome.

Longevity: Studies suggest that adhering to the Mediterranean Diet is associated with increased life expectancy. The combination of nutrient-rich foods and a lifestyle that includes physical activity and social connections contributes to overall longevity.

Principles guiding a Mediterranean Diet Cookbook incorporate these health benefits by offering recipes that align with the core elements of the diet. These recipes often emphasize the use of fresh, seasonal ingredients, mindful cooking techniques, and the celebration of diverse flavors. By embracing these principles, individuals can not only enjoy delicious meals but also foster a sustainable and health-promoting way of life inspired by the Mediterranean tradition.

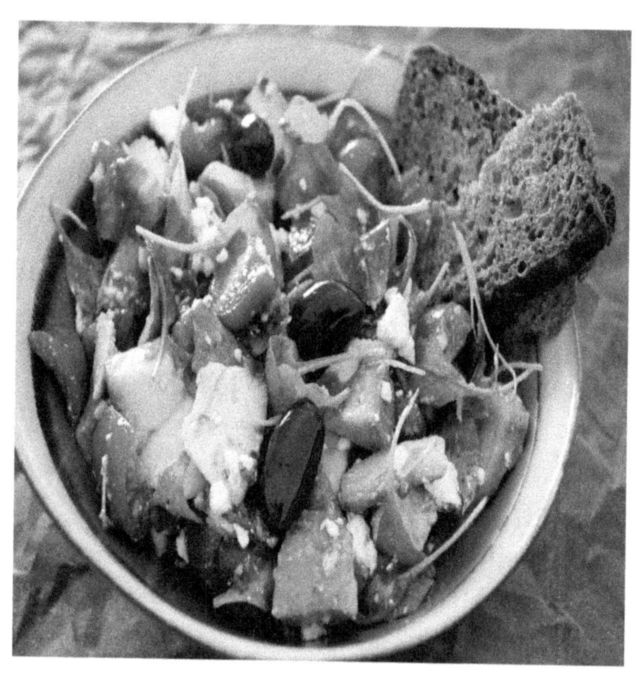

CHAPTER TWO

2 Getting Started

"Getting Started" with the Mediterranean Diet Cookbook for beginners is a crucial section that lays the foundation for a successful journey into this vibrant and healthful way of eating. This section serves as a practical guide, offering essential information and tips to seamlessly integrate the Mediterranean Diet into daily life.

Kitchen Essentials:
Olive Oil: Highlight the importance of using extra virgin olive oil as a primary source of healthy fats.
Herbs and Spices: Encourage the use of Mediterranean herbs and spices to enhance flavors without relying on excessive salt or unhealthy condiments.

Whole Grains: Stock up on whole grains like quinoa, bulgur, and brown rice for a diverse and nutritious carbohydrate base.

Grocery Shopping Guide:
Produce Section: Guide beginners through selecting a variety of colorful fruits and vegetables to ensure a rich spectrum of nutrients.
Seafood Choices: Educate on choosing sustainable fish and seafood options, emphasizing their omega-3 fatty acid content.
Lean Proteins: Include lean protein sources like poultry, beans, and legumes, promoting a balance between plant and animal-based proteins.

Meal Planning Tips:
Balanced Meals: Emphasize the importance of creating balanced meals that include a variety of food groups, such as vegetables, whole grains, and lean proteins.

Portion Control: Provide guidance on portion sizes to help beginners maintain a healthy caloric intake.

Snack Options: Suggest wholesome snack ideas, such as nuts, fruits, or Greek yogurt, to keep energy levels stable between meals.

Culinary Techniques:

Grilling and Roasting: Encourage cooking methods like grilling and roasting to preserve the nutritional value of ingredients while enhancing flavors.

Minimal Processing: Advocate for minimal processing of ingredients to retain their natural goodness and health benefits.

Mediterranean Pantry Staples:

Canned Tomatoes: Discuss the versatility and convenience of canned tomatoes in Mediterranean cooking.

Legumes: Highlight the significance of incorporating legumes like chickpeas and lentils for protein and fiber.

Exploring Mediterranean Flavors:
Citrus Fruits: Introduce the zesty and refreshing flavors of citrus fruits like lemons and oranges.
Feta and Olives: Explore the savory delights of feta cheese and olives, adding unique Mediterranean touches to dishes.

By delving into the "Getting Started" section, beginners are equipped with the knowledge and tools needed to navigate the Mediterranean Diet with confidence. This practical foundation sets the stage for an enjoyable and healthful culinary experience, making the transition into this lifestyle both seamless and gratifying.

2.1 Kitchen Essentials

Creating delicious and wholesome Mediterranean-inspired meals starts with having the right tools and ingredients in your kitchen. This "Kitchen Essentials" section serves as a guide for beginners, helping them stock their kitchens with items that are fundamental to the preparation of authentic and nutritious Mediterranean dishes.

Extra Virgin Olive Oil (EVOO):
Importance: Emphasize the central role of EVOO in Mediterranean cooking for its heart-healthy monounsaturated fats and rich flavor.
Usage: Teach proper storing and drizzling techniques, as EVOO is a staple in dressings, marinades, and sautéing.

Herbs and Spices:
Mediterranean Herbs: Include essentials like oregano, thyme, rosemary, and basil to add depth and aroma to dishes.
Spice Blends: Introduce popular blends like za'atar or de Provence for a burst of Mediterranean flavor.

Whole Grains:
Quinoa, Bulgur, Farro: Explain the versatility of these grains as a base for salads, pilafs, or sides, providing fiber and essential nutrients.

Canned Tomatoes:
Versatility: Discuss the convenience of canned tomatoes for sauces, soups, and stews, emphasizing the importance of choosing high-quality options.

Legumes:
Chickpeas, Lentils, and Beans: Showcase legumes as protein-rich alternatives, perfect for salads, dips, or hearty stews.

Seafood:
Frozen or Fresh: Advise on keeping frozen seafood for convenience and fresh options for a delightful variety of flavors.
Anchovies and Sardines: Introduce these flavorful additions, commonly used in Mediterranean cuisine.

Lean Proteins:
Chicken and Turkey: Promote the inclusion of lean poultry as a primary protein source.
Greek Yogurt: Emphasize its versatility in both savory and sweet dishes, providing a rich source of protein and probiotics.

Nuts and Seeds:
Almonds, Walnuts, Chia Seeds: Discuss their role in adding crunch and nutritional value to salads, yogurts, or desserts.

Fruits and Vegetables:
Tomatoes, Eggplants, Zucchini: Highlight the abundant use of fresh produce in Mediterranean cooking for vibrant colors and essential nutrients.
Citrus Fruits: Incorporate lemons and oranges for zesty flavors in both savory and sweet dishes.

Whole Wheat Pasta and Brown Rice:
Healthy Alternatives: Introduce whole grain options, emphasizing their higher fiber content and nutritional benefits.

By familiarizing themselves with these kitchen essentials, beginners are well-equipped to dive into the world of Mediterranean cooking with confidence. These foundational ingredients pave the way for a diverse and healthful culinary experience that captures the essence of this renowned and time-tested dietary tradition.

2.2 **Grocery Shopping Guide**

Navigating the aisles with a clear understanding of what to include in your grocery cart is essential for success in adopting the Mediterranean Diet. This detailed guide for beginners ensures that your shopping list aligns with the principles of this healthful and flavorful culinary tradition.

Fresh Produce Section:
Colorful Vegetables: Prioritize a variety of colorful vegetables such as tomatoes, bell peppers, spinach, and kale for their rich nutrient profiles.
Seasonal Fruits: Choose a selection of seasonal fruits like berries, citrus fruits, and melons for natural sweetness and antioxidants.

Seafood Choices:
Fatty Fish: Opt for fatty fish like salmon, mackerel, and sardines, rich in omega-3 fatty acids for heart health.
Shellfish: Include options like shrimp and mussels for variety and additional protein sources.

Lean Proteins:
Poultry: Select lean poultry options like chicken or turkey breasts, suitable for grilling, roasting, or sautéing.
Legumes: Stock up on chickpeas, lentils, and various beans for plant-based protein and fiber.

Whole Grains:
Quinoa, Bulgur, Farro: Include these versatile whole grains to serve as the base for salads, side dishes, or main courses.
Whole Wheat Pasta and Brown Rice: Choose whole grain alternatives for added fiber and nutritional benefits.

Dairy and Alternatives:
Greek Yogurt: Opt for Greek yogurt for its thick texture and higher protein content.
Feta and Parmesan Cheese: Enhance flavors with these cheeses in moderation, adding richness to salads and dishes.

Canned and Jarred Goods:
Canned Tomatoes: Choose high-quality canned tomatoes for sauces, soups, and stews.
Olives and Capers: Add briny flavors to your dishes with various types of olives and capers.

Nuts and Seeds:
Almonds, Walnuts, Chia Seeds: Include a mix of nuts and seeds for snacking or adding crunch to salads and yogurts.

Herbs and Spices:
Oregano, Thyme, Rosemary: Pick up these Mediterranean herbs for aromatic and flavorful dishes.
Spice Blends: Explore blends like za'atar or de Provence for an authentic taste.

Olive Oil:
Extra Virgin Olive Oil: Invest in high-quality extra virgin olive oil for cooking, dressing, and drizzling.

Bakery Section:
Whole Grain Breads and Pitas: Look for whole grain options for sandwiches or dipping into olive oil.

Frozen Section:
Frozen Vegetables and Fruits: Keep a stock of frozen options for convenience without compromising nutritional value.
Frozen Fish: Consider keeping frozen fish for quick and easy protein sources.

Heritage and Ethnic Aisles:

Mediterranean Ingredients: Explore specialty aisles for unique Mediterranean ingredients like tahini, couscous, or pomegranate molasses.

By following this comprehensive Grocery Shopping Guide, beginners can fill their carts with nutrient-dense, flavorful ingredients, setting the stage for a successful and enjoyable journey into the Mediterranean Diet.

2.3 Meal Planning Tips

Effective meal planning is key to successfully adopting the Mediterranean Diet. These tips provide beginners with practical guidance on structuring their meals to align with the principles of this wholesome and flavorful way of eating.

Balanced Meals:
Incorporate All Food Groups: Aim for well-rounded meals that include a variety of vegetables, fruits, whole grains, lean proteins, and healthy fats.
Colorful Plate: Strive for a colorful plate, indicating a diverse range of nutrients and antioxidants.

Mindful Portions: Controlling Portion Size
Make mindful eating a habit by paying attention to portion proportions. Rather than overindulging, concentrate on expressing your hunger.
Make Use of Smaller Plates: Select smaller plates to facilitate organic portion control.

Snack Smart:
Wholesome Snacking: Choose nutrient-dense snacks such as nuts, fresh fruits, or Greek yogurt to curb hunger between meals.
Preparation is Key: Prepare snack-sized portions in advance to avoid reaching for less nutritious options.

Regular Meals and Snacks:
Consistent Eating Schedule: Establish a regular eating schedule with balanced meals and planned snacks to maintain energy levels throughout the day.
Avoid Skipping Meals: Avoid skipping meals to prevent excessive hunger and overeating later in the day.

Mediterranean Breakfast Ideas:
Greek Yogurt Parfait: Layer Greek yogurt with fresh fruits, nuts, and a drizzle of honey for a nutrient-packed breakfast.
Mediterranean Omelette: Include tomatoes, spinach, feta, and olives for a flavorful and satisfying start to the day.

Lunch and Dinner Inspiration:
Quinoa Greek Salad: Prepare a hearty salad with quinoa, cherry tomatoes, cucumber, feta, and a lemon vinaigrette.
Baked Mediterranean Chicken: Season chicken with herbs, garlic, and olive oil, and bake for a delicious and protein-rich dinner.

Meal Prep for Convenience:
Batch Cooking: Prepare batches of grains, legumes, and proteins at the beginning of the week for quick and easy meal assembly.
Chop Veggies in Advance: Save time by chopping vegetables in advance, making it convenient to add them to various dishes.

Hydration:
Water and Herbal Teas: Prioritize hydration with water and herbal teas. Limit sugary drinks and excessive caffeine.
Infused Water: Enhance water with citrus slices, mint, or cucumber for a refreshing twist.

Dessert Choices:
Fresh Fruit Desserts: Opt for fresh fruits, like berries or citrus, for a naturally sweet and healthful dessert.
Moderation with Sweets: If craving sweets, choose small portions of desserts made with wholesome ingredients.

Explore New Recipes:
Variety is Key: Keep meals exciting by exploring new recipes from the cookbook, trying different ingredients, and experimenting with Mediterranean flavors.

CHAPTER THREE

3 Core Components of the Mediterranean Diet

The Mediterranean Diet is characterized by a rich tapestry of fresh, nutrient-dense foods that contribute to its reputation as a heart-healthy and balanced way of eating. Understanding the core components is key to adopting this lifestyle successfully.

Fruits and Vegetables:
Abundance: Fill your plate with a rainbow of fruits and vegetables, aiming for at least 5 servings per day.
Seasonal Choices: Emphasize seasonal produce for optimal freshness and flavor.
Raw and Cooked: Enjoy a mix of raw and cooked vegetables to maximize nutrient intake.

Whole Grains:
Diverse Options: Incorporate a variety of whole grains such as whole wheat, barley, quinoa, and brown rice.
Fiber-Rich: Whole grains provide essential fiber, promoting digestive health and satiety.
Balanced Carbohydrates: Opt for complex carbohydrates, which release energy slowly, supporting stable blood sugar levels.

Healthy Fats:
Extra Virgin Olive Oil (EVOO): Make EVOO your primary source of fat for its monounsaturated fats and antioxidant properties.
Nuts and Seeds: Include almonds, walnuts, chia seeds, and flaxseeds for additional healthy fats and omega-3 fatty acids.
Fatty Fish: Regularly consume fish like salmon and mackerel for omega-3s, benefiting heart and brain health.

Lean Proteins:
Poultry: Choose lean cuts of chicken and turkey, and remove skin to minimize saturated fat intake.
Legumes: Incorporate beans, lentils, and chickpeas as excellent plant-based protein sources.
Moderate Red Meat: Consume red meat in moderation, opting for lean cuts and limiting processed meats.

Dairy and Alternatives:
Greek Yogurt and Cheese: Choose Greek yogurt for its higher protein content and include moderate amounts of feta or Parmesan for added flavor.
Limited Dairy: Consume dairy in moderation, considering alternatives like plant-based milk or yogurt if preferred.

Fruits as Desserts:
Natural Sweetness: Let fresh fruits serve as desserts, providing natural sweetness and an array of vitamins and minerals.
Dried Fruits: Occasionally include dried fruits like dates or figs for a sweet treat in moderation.

Herbs and Spices:
Flavorful Seasoning: Use herbs like oregano, thyme, rosemary, and spices like cumin and paprika to enhance flavors without excessive salt.
Mediterranean Blends: Explore traditional spice blends such as za'atar for an authentic touch.

Wine in Moderation:
Occasional Enjoyment: If you choose to drink alcohol, do so in moderation, with red wine being a common choice for its potential heart benefits.
Hydration: Prioritize water as the primary beverage to stay well-hydrated.

3.1 **Fruits and Vegetables**

Fruits and vegetables are the vibrant stars of the Mediterranean Diet, providing a spectrum of flavors, nutrients, and health benefits. In the cookbook for beginners, the emphasis on these fresh and colorful ingredients is foundational to creating delicious and nourishing meals.

Abundance and Variety:
Daily Intake: Encourage a daily intake of at least 5 servings of fruits and vegetables, emphasizing variety for a broad range of nutrients.
Diverse Colors: Highlight the importance of including fruits and vegetables of various colors to ensure a mix of vitamins, minerals, and antioxidants.

Seasonal Choices:
Freshness and Flavor: Emphasize the use of seasonal produce for optimal freshness and flavor. This also supports local and sustainable eating.
Seasonal Recipes: Introduce seasonal recipes that showcase the best fruits and vegetables available during different times of the year.

Raw and Cooked Options:
Raw for Crunch and Nutrients: Promote the consumption of raw vegetables for added crunch and to preserve maximum nutrient content.
Cooked for Versatility: Highlight the versatility of cooked vegetables, which can be roasted, grilled, steamed, or sautéed to enhance flavors and textures.

Key Vegetables:
Tomatoes: A Mediterranean staple, rich in antioxidants and used in sauces, salads, and various dishes.

Eggplants: Versatile and often used in dishes like ratatouille or grilled for a smoky flavor. Zucchini and Bell Peppers: Commonly used in salads, stir-fries, or stuffed recipes, adding color and nutrients.

Key Fruits:
Citrus Fruits: Oranges, lemons, and grapefruits provide zesty flavors and are rich in vitamin C.
Berries: Strawberries, blueberries, and raspberries contribute natural sweetness and antioxidants.
Apples and Pears: Ideal for snacking or incorporating into salads and desserts.

Incorporating Fruits into Meals:
Breakfast Ideas: Encourage adding sliced fruits to Greek yogurt, blending them into smoothies, or enjoying them with whole grain cereals.
Lunch and Dinner: Showcase recipes that incorporate fruits into savory dishes, such as fruit salads, salsas, or chutneys served with grilled proteins.

Vegetarian and Plant-Based Options:
Vegetarian Main Courses: Introduce recipes where vegetables take center stage, such as stuffed bell peppers, vegetable gratins, or roasted cauliflower steaks.
Plant-Based Meals: Showcase the abundance of plant-based options, emphasizing legumes, whole grains, and a colorful array of vegetables in salads or Buddha bowls.

Snacking and Desserts:
Fresh Snacking: Encourage fresh fruits as convenient and nutritious snacks.
Dessert Alternatives: Suggest desserts that feature fruits, such as fruit salads, poached fruits, or simple fruit sorbets.

Tips for Storage and Preparation:
Proper Storage: Guide beginners on proper storage to maximize the shelf life of fruits and vegetables.
Easy Prep Techniques: Include simple and quick preparation techniques, like chopping, slicing, or marinating, to make incorporating these ingredients seamless.

By exploring the rich world of fruits and vegetables in the Mediterranean Diet Cookbook for Beginners, individuals can unlock the potential for creating vibrant, flavorful, and healthful meals that celebrate the essence of this iconic culinary tradition.

3.2 **Whole Grains**

In the context of the Mediterranean diet, Whole Grains constitute a cornerstone, providing a plethora of health benefits and culinary versatility. This comprehensive overview explores the significance, types, and incorporation of whole grains within the framework of this renowned dietary pattern.

Diversity of Whole Grains:
Quinoa: A protein-rich grain with a complete amino acid profile, suitable for salads and side dishes.
Bulgur: Quick-cooking and fiber-packed, often used in traditional Mediterranean dishes like tabbouleh.
Farro: Nutrient-dense and chewy, adding a hearty texture to salads and soups.
Brown Rice: Retains bran and germ layers, offering a wholesome base for various

Mediterranean recipes.

Barley: Rich in fiber and vitamins, contributing to heart health and frequently incorporated into soups.

Nutritional Benefits:

Abundant in fiber, whole grains support digestive health and provide a sustained energy release.

Rich in essential nutrients such as vitamins, minerals, and antioxidants, contributing to overall well-being.

Low glycemic index, aiding in blood sugar control and weight management.

Culinary Integration:

Salads: Whole grains enhance the texture and nutritional content of salads, creating filling and satisfying meals.

Pilafs: Incorporated into traditional Mediterranean rice dishes, adding a nutrient-rich dimension.

Breads and Pastas: Whole grain varieties offer alternatives to refined grains in Mediterranean cuisine.

Cooking Techniques:
Detailed instructions on cooking methods, ensuring optimal flavor and texture.
Emphasis on minimizing processing to retain the nutritional integrity of grains.

Balancing Act:
Guidance on portion control to maintain balance within the Mediterranean diet.
Integration with other diet components such as fresh vegetables, lean proteins, and healthy fats.

Health Implications:
by lowering the risk of cardiovascular illnesses, promotes heart health.
improves satiety and nutrient density to aid with weight management.

sustains energy, which is essential for the active lifestyle that is frequently connected to the Mediterranean region.

Practical Tips:
Shopping guides for selecting high-quality whole grains.
Tips on storing and incorporating whole grains into everyday meals.
In essence, Whole Grains in the Mediterranean diet serve as nutritional powerhouses, promoting health and flavor in equal measure. This comprehensive understanding empowers individuals to embrace these grains as integral components of a balanced and wholesome Mediterranean eating pattern.

3.3 Healthy Fats

Healthy fats play a pivotal role in the Mediterranean diet, contributing to both culinary richness and numerous health benefits. This comprehensive exploration elucidates the types, sources, and health implications of healthy fats within the context of the Mediterranean diet.

Olive Oil:
Monounsaturated Fat: Predominantly found in olive oil, this heart-healthy fat is a cornerstone of the Mediterranean diet.
Extra Virgin Olive Oil: Unrefined and rich in antioxidants, contributing to cardiovascular health.

Nuts and Seeds:
Polyunsaturated Fats: Present in abundance in nuts and seeds.

Omega-3 Fatty Acids: Particularly in walnuts and flaxseeds, supporting brain health and reducing inflammation.

Fatty Fish:
Omega-3 Fatty Acids: Abundant in fish like salmon, mackerel, and sardines.
Heart Health: Supports cardiovascular health and reduces the risk of chronic diseases.

Avocado:
Monounsaturated Fat: Similar to olive oil, avocados provide a creamy texture and heart-healthy fats.
Nutrient Density: Rich in vitamins, minerals, and fiber, enhancing overall nutritional intake.

Cheese and Yogurt:
Saturated Fats in Moderation: Dairy in the Mediterranean diet is often consumed in moderation, providing essential nutrients.

Calcium and Protein: Dairy contributes to bone health and satiety.

Balancing Fats in the Diet:
Portion Control: Emphasis on moderation to maintain overall caloric balance.
Replacing Saturated Fats: Substituting saturated fats with monounsaturated and polyunsaturated fats for heart health.

Cooking Techniques:
Olive Oil as a Culinary Staple: Used for sautéing, dressing, and as a flavor enhancer.
Grilling and Baking: Preferred methods to retain nutritional integrity while enhancing flavors.

Health Implications:
Cardiovascular Health: Monounsaturated and polyunsaturated fats contribute to lower cholesterol levels and reduced risk of heart disease.

Brain Health: Omega-3 fatty acids support cognitive function and may reduce the risk of neurodegenerative diseases.

Practical Tips:
Choosing High-Quality Oils: Guidance on selecting extra virgin olive oil and other quality fats.
Incorporating Variety: Encouragement to include a variety of healthy fats for a well-rounded diet.

In essence, understanding healthy fats in the Mediterranean diet involves recognizing the synergy between culinary enjoyment and health promotion. By embracing a diverse array of fats from plant-based sources and seafood, individuals can optimize their nutrition and overall well-being within the framework of this renowned dietary pattern.

3.4 Lean Proteins

Lean proteins are an essential component of the Mediterranean diet, providing a source of high-quality nutrition without excess saturated fats. This comprehensive overview explores the types, sources, and health implications of lean proteins within the context of the Mediterranean diet.

Poultry:

Chicken and Turkey: Lean sources of protein, versatile for various Mediterranean dishes.

Grilled or Roasted: Cooking methods that retain nutritional value without adding excessive fats.

Fish and Seafood:

Fatty Fish: Such as salmon, mackerel, and sardines provide omega-3 fatty acids.

Lean Choices: Options like cod and haddock are rich in protein and low in saturated fats.

Legumes:
Beans and Lentils: Excellent plant-based sources of protein, fiber, and various nutrients.
Versatility: Suitable for salads, stews, and side dishes.

Lean Cuts of Meat:
Pork and Beef: Opting for lean cuts, such as loin or sirloin, reduces saturated fat intake.
Grass-fed Options: Healthier fat profile compared to conventionally raised meat.

Eggs:
Protein-Rich: Eggs are a versatile and nutrient-dense protein source.
Moderation: Consuming eggs in moderation aligns with the balanced approach of the Mediterranean diet.

Dairy:
Low-Fat or Fat-Free Options: Choosing yogurt and cheese with reduced fat content. Greek Yogurt: High in protein and a staple in the Mediterranean diet.

Plant-Based Proteins:
Nuts and Seeds: Adding protein and healthy fats to meals and snacks.
Tofu and Tempeh: Suitable meat alternatives with added nutritional benefits.

Cooking Techniques:
Grilling and Baking: Methods that preserve the leanness of proteins without excessive added fats.
Herbs and Spices: Flavoring proteins with herbs and spices reduces the reliance on heavy sauces.

Health Implications:
Muscle Health: Adequate protein intake supports muscle maintenance and repair.
Weight Management: Lean proteins contribute to a feeling of fullness, aiding in weight control.

Practical Tips:
Balanced Meals: Incorporating lean proteins with a variety of vegetables and whole grains.
Mindful Cooking: Limiting the use of frying and choosing healthier cooking methods.

In summary, lean proteins in the Mediterranean diet contribute to overall health by providing essential nutrients while aligning with the principles of moderation and balance. Integrating a variety of lean protein sources ensures a diverse and satisfying approach to this renowned dietary pattern.

3.5 Dairy and Alternatives

In the Mediterranean diet, dairy and its alternatives are incorporated in a balanced manner, providing essential nutrients while mindful of overall health. This comprehensive overview explores the types, sources, and health implications of dairy and dairy alternatives within the context of the Mediterranean diet.

Dairy:
Yogurt: Greek yogurt, in particular, is a staple, offering protein, probiotics, and essential nutrients.
Cheese: Moderation is key, with an emphasis on flavorful, aged varieties.
Milk: Often consumed in smaller amounts, with a preference for low-fat or skim options.

Plant-Based Alternatives:
Almond Milk, Soy Milk, and Oat Milk:
Provide alternatives for those avoiding dairy.
Nutritional Content: Fortified varieties offer
essential vitamins and minerals.

Nutritional Benefits:
Calcium and Vitamin D: Vital for bone health,
with dairy and fortified alternatives contributing
to daily requirements.
Protein: Dairy, especially Greek yogurt, is a
notable source of high-quality protein.
Probiotics: Found in yogurt, supporting gut
health.

Moderation and Balance:
Portion Control: Enjoying dairy in moderate
amounts aligns with the Mediterranean diet's
balanced approach.
Reduced-Fat Options: Choosing low-fat or
fat-free dairy options for heart health.

Culinary Integration:
Yogurt in Cooking: Utilizing yogurt as a versatile ingredient in both savory and sweet Mediterranean dishes.
Cheese as Flavor Enhancer: Incorporating small amounts of flavorful cheeses to add richness to meals.

Plant-Based Proteins:
Tofu and Tempeh: Offering protein and serving as alternatives for those opting for plant-based sources.
Nuts and Seeds: Providing additional protein and healthy fats.

Lactose Sensitivity:
Lactose-Free Options: For individuals with lactose intolerance, lactose-free dairy or plant-based alternatives offer suitable choices.

Health Implications:
Bone Health: Dairy and fortified alternatives contribute to calcium intake, crucial for bone strength.
Heart Health: Choosing lower-fat dairy options supports cardiovascular well-being.

Practical Tips:
Label Reading: Checking labels for added sugars in flavored dairy alternatives.
Homemade Options: Making plant-based milk alternatives at home for control over ingredients.

In essence, incorporating dairy and its alternatives in the Mediterranean diet involves a balanced approach, emphasizing nutrient-rich options in moderate quantities. This inclusive perspective allows individuals to enjoy the culinary richness of dairy while accommodating preferences and dietary considerations within the context of this renowned eating pattern.

CHAPTER FOUR

4 Flavorful Herbs and Spices

The Mediterranean diet is renowned for its rich flavors, and herbs and spices play a crucial role in achieving that delicious taste. Here are some key flavorful herbs and spices commonly used in the Mediterranean diet:

Basil: Adds a sweet and slightly peppery flavor, often used in tomato-based dishes, salads, and pasta.

Oregano: A staple in Mediterranean cuisine, it has a robust, earthy flavor. It's used in various dishes, including pizzas, salads, and grilled meats.

Rosemary: Known for its pine-like aroma, it pairs well with roasted vegetables, lamb, and poultry.

Thyme: Offers a subtle earthy taste and is frequently used in stews, soups, and grilled dishes.

Parsley: Provides a fresh and slightly peppery flavor, commonly used as a garnish or in salads, sauces, and marinades.

Mint: Adds a refreshing touch, often used in salads, teas, and desserts.

Garlic: A fundamental ingredient, it adds a strong and savory flavor to various dishes.

Cumin: Although more associated with Middle Eastern cuisine, it's used in Mediterranean dishes, providing a warm and slightly nutty flavor.

Coriander: Commonly used in Mediterranean spice blends, it contributes a citrusy and slightly sweet taste.

Paprika: Adds a mild, sweet, or smoky flavor, enhancing dishes like stews, soups, and grilled meats.

Fennel: With a mild licorice taste, it's often used in salads and to flavor fish dishes.

Saffron: A luxurious spice, it imparts a distinctive earthy and slightly bitter taste, used in paella and various rice dishes.

Combining these herbs and spices allows for a diverse and flavorful culinary experience, characteristic of the Mediterranean diet.

4.1 Common Mediterranean Herbs

Here's a detailed explanation of some common Mediterranean herbs:

Basil:
Flavor Profile: Sweet, slightly peppery.
Common Uses: Pesto, salads, pasta, tomato-based dishes.

Oregano:
Flavor Profile: Robust, earthy.
Common Uses: Pizzas, salads, grilled meats, Mediterranean sauces.

Rosemary:
Flavor Profile: Pine-like aroma, slightly woody.
Common Uses: Roasted vegetables, lamb, poultry, marinades.

Thyme:
Flavor Profile: Subtle earthy taste.
Common Uses: Stews, soups, grilled dishes, roasted meats.

Parsley:
Flavor Profile: Fresh, slightly peppery.
Common Uses: Garnish, salads, sauces, marinades, Mediterranean tabbouleh.

Mint:
Flavor Profile: Refreshing.
Common Uses: Salads, teas, desserts, lamb dishes.

Garlic:
Flavor Profile: Strong, savory.
Common Uses: Almost all savory dishes, Mediterranean dips, sauces.

Cumin:
Flavor Profile: Warm, slightly nutty.
Common Uses: Spice blends, roasted vegetables, grains.

Coriander:
Flavor Profile: Citrusy, slightly sweet.
Common Uses: Spice blends, marinades, couscous.

Paprika:
Flavor Profile: Mild, sweet, or smoky.
Common Uses: Stews, soups, grilled meats, Mediterranean rice dishes.

Fennel:
Flavor Profile: Mild licorice taste.
Common Uses: Salads, fish dishes, roasted vegetables.

Saffron:

Flavor Profile: Distinctive, earthy, slightly bitter.

Common Uses: Paella, rice dishes, sauces.

These herbs contribute not only to the flavor but also to the aromatic and vibrant character of Mediterranean cuisine, creating a unique and delightful culinary experience.

4.2 **Spice Blends for Authentic Flavors**

Creating authentic Mediterranean flavors often involves the use of spice blends that capture the essence of the region. Here are some common spice blends used in the Mediterranean diet:

Herbes de Provence:
Ingredients: Typically a mix of dried thyme, rosemary, oregano, marjoram, and sometimes lavender.
Common Uses: Roasted vegetables, grilled meats, stews, and Mediterranean-style roasted chicken.

Za'atar:
Ingredients: Thyme, sesame seeds, sumac, and salt.
Common Uses: Sprinkled on flatbreads, used in marinades, as a seasoning for salads or grilled meats.

Ras el Hanout:
Ingredients: A complex blend that may include cinnamon, cumin, coriander, ginger, cardamom, nutmeg, and more.
Common Uses: Tagines, couscous dishes, roasted vegetables, and grilled meats.

Baharat:
Ingredients: A blend of black pepper, cumin, coriander, cinnamon, cloves, and nutmeg.
Common Uses: Seasoning for lamb, beef, and chicken, as well as in rice and lentil dishes.

Italian Seasoning:
Ingredients: Typically a mix of dried basil, oregano, rosemary, thyme, and sometimes garlic powder.
Common Uses: Pasta sauces, pizzas, salads, and roasted vegetables.

Greek Seasoning:
Ingredients: Often includes dried oregano, mint, garlic powder, onion powder, and sometimes dill.
Common Uses: Grilled meats, Greek salads, roasted vegetables, and Mediterranean-style marinades.

Harissa Spice Blend:
Ingredients: Ground chili peppers, garlic, coriander, caraway, and cumin.
Common Uses: Adding heat and flavor to stews, couscous, grilled meats, and roasted vegetables.

Sumac Spice Blend:
Ingredients: Mainly sumac, sometimes mixed with sesame seeds and thyme.
Common Uses: Sprinkled on salads, grilled meats, and as a seasoning for Middle Eastern dishes.

Cretan Blend (Mediterranean Island Blend):
Ingredients: A mix of oregano, thyme, rosemary, and sometimes dried citrus zest.
Common Uses: Seasoning for grilled fish, roasted vegetables, and Mediterranean-style soups.

Advieh:
Ingredients: Commonly a combination of cinnamon, nutmeg, cardamom, and dried rose petals.
Common Uses: Persian-influenced dishes, rice pilafs, and as a rub for grilled meats.

These spice blends add depth, complexity, and authenticity to Mediterranean dishes, enhancing the overall culinary experience.

CHAPTER FIVE

5 Delicious Recipes

Greek salad topped with grilled chicken:
Components:
Various greens
rosy tomatoes
Cucumbers
crimson onions
Olives kalamata
Feta cheese
A grilled chicken breast
Lemon dressing with olive oil
Guidelines:
In a big bowl, toss together the mixed greens, tomatoes, cucumbers, red onions, olives, and feta.
Add some grilled chicken slices on top.
Drizzle with a dressing consisting of lemon juice, olive oil, salt, and pepper.

Mediterranean Stuffed Peppers:
Ingredients:
Bell peppers
Quinoa
Chickpeas
Cherry tomatoes
Feta cheese
Fresh parsley
Olive oil, garlic, and lemon juice
Instructions:
Cook quinoa and mix with chickpeas, diced
tomatoes, feta, chopped parsley, olive oil,
garlic, and lemon juice.
Cut bell peppers in half, remove seeds, and
stuff with the quinoa mixture.
Bake until peppers are tender.

Grilled Mediterranean Vegetables:
Ingredients:
Zucchini
Eggplant
Bell peppers
Cherry tomatoes
Red onion
Olive oil, balsamic vinegar, and herbs
(rosemary, thyme)
Instructions:
Cut vegetables into bite-sized pieces.
Toss with olive oil, balsamic vinegar, and
herbs.
Grill until vegetables are tender and slightly
charred.

Mediterranean Baked Fish:
Ingredients:
White fish filets (e.g., cod or tilapia)
Cherry tomatoes
Kalamata olives
Capers
Garlic

Olive oil, lemon juice, and fresh herbs (parsley, oregano)
Instructions:
Place fish filets in a baking dish.
Top with halved cherry tomatoes, olives, capers, and minced garlic.
Drizzle with olive oil and lemon juice, then bake until the fish flakes easily.
Garnish with fresh herbs before serving.

Ingredients for a Mediterranean Chickpea Salad: chickpeas
rosy tomatoes
Cucumbers
Onion red
Feta cheese
Olives kalamata
Red wine vinegar and olive oil
new oregano

Guidelines:
In a bowl, mix together chickpeas, tomatoes, cucumbers, red onion, feta, and olives.
Add a drizzle of red wine vinegar and olive oil.
Add some fresh oregano and mix everything together.

Mediterranean Grilled Shrimp Skewers:
Ingredients:
Large shrimp, peeled and deveined
Cherry tomatoes
Red and yellow bell peppers, cut into chunks
Red onion, cut into wedges
Olive oil, lemon juice, garlic, oregano
Instructions:
Marinate shrimp and vegetables in a mixture of olive oil, lemon juice, minced garlic, and oregano.
Thread onto skewers and grill until shrimp are opaque and vegetables are tender.

Eggplant and Tomato Bake:
Ingredients:
Eggplant, sliced
Tomatoes, sliced
Garlic, minced
Fresh basil and oregano
Olive oil
Parmesan cheese
Instructions:
Layer sliced eggplant and tomatoes in a baking
dish.
Drizzle with olive oil, sprinkle with minced
garlic, fresh herbs, and Parmesan.
Bake until bubbly and golden.

Mediterranean Quinoa Bowl:
Ingredients:
Cooked quinoa
Chickpeas
Spinach or kale
Cherry tomatoes, halved
Cucumber, diced
Feta cheese

Kalamata olives
Olive oil and lemon dressing
Instructions:
Assemble a bowl with quinoa as the base, then
arrange chickpeas, vegetables, feta, and
olives.
Drizzle with olive oil and lemon dressing.

Greek Chicken Souvlaki:
Ingredients:
Chicken breast, cut into cubes
Greek yogurt
Lemon juice, garlic, oregano
Cucumber, tomatoes, red onion
Pita bread
Instructions:
Marinate chicken in Greek yogurt, lemon juice,
minced garlic, and oregano.
Thread onto skewers and grill.
Serve in pita with chopped vegetables and a
dollop of tzatziki.

Mediterranean Lentil Soup:
Ingredients:
Green or brown lentils
Carrots, celery, onion
Garlic, tomatoes
Spinach or kale
Olive oil, cumin, coriander, thyme
Instructions:
Sauté vegetables in olive oil until softened.
Add lentils, tomatoes, and spices; simmer until lentils are tender.
Stir in fresh greens before serving.

These recipes showcase the diversity of Mediterranean cuisine, incorporating a variety of fresh and wholesome ingredients. Whether you prefer seafood, vegetables, or lean meats, these dishes provide a delicious and nutritious way to embrace the Mediterranean diet.

5.1 **Breakfast**

Greek Yogurt with Honey and Fresh Fruit:
Ingredients:
Greek yogurt
Honey
Fresh fruits (berries, figs, or sliced peaches)
Optional: Nuts (like almonds or walnuts)
Instructions:
Spoon Greek yogurt into a bowl.
Drizzle with honey.
Top with a variety of fresh fruits and a sprinkle
of nuts for added texture.

Mediterranean Omelette:
Ingredients:
Eggs
Cherry tomatoes, diced
Spinach
Feta cheese
Olives, sliced
Olive oil

Instructions:
Whisk eggs and pour into a heated pan with olive oil.
Add diced tomatoes, spinach, feta, and olives.
Cook until eggs are set, then fold the omelet.

Toast made of whole grains, avocado, and **poached egg:**
Ingredients: Toasted Ripe avocado, whole grain bread
a stolen egg
Sliced cherry tomatoes
Fresh herbs, such as chives or parsley
Guidelines:
Toast the whole grain bread and spread the avocado spread.
Add sliced cherry tomatoes and a poached egg on top.
Add some fresh herb garnish.

Mediterranean Smoothie Bowl:
Ingredients:
Greek yogurt
Mixed berries
Banana
Spinach or kale
Chia seeds
Honey
Instructions:
Blend Greek yogurt, mixed berries, banana,
and greens until smooth.
Pour into a bowl and top with chia seeds and a
drizzle of honey.

Mediterranean Breakfast Wrap:
Ingredients:
Whole grain tortilla
Hummus
Sliced cucumber and tomatoes
Feta cheese
Olives, chopped

Instructions:
Spread hummus on a whole grain tortilla.
Layer with sliced cucumber, tomatoes, feta,
and chopped olives.
Roll into a wrap and enjoy.

Mediterranean Baked Eggs:
Ingredients:
Eggs
Tomatoes, diced
Bell peppers, diced
Red onion, chopped
Feta cheese
Fresh oregano
Instructions:
Preheat the oven and bake cracked eggs over
a bed of diced tomatoes, peppers, and onions.
Crumble feta over the eggs and sprinkle with
fresh oregano.

5.2 **Lunch**

Mediterranean Chickpea Salad: Ingredients:
chopped Feta cheese, crumbled Kalamata
olives, diced red onion, cooked cherry
tomatoes, chopped cucumber, sliced olive oil,
and red wine vinegar dressing
Parsley or oregano fresh
Guidelines:
Chickpeas, tomatoes, cucumbers, red onions,
feta, and olives should all be combined in a
bowl.
Add a drizzle of red wine vinegar and olive oil.
Add some fresh herb garnish.

Greek Quinoa Salad:
Ingredients:
Quinoa, cooked
Cherry tomatoes, halved
Cucumber, diced
Red bell pepper, chopped
Red onion, finely sliced
Feta cheese, crumbled

Kalamata olives, sliced
Olive oil, lemon juice, and oregano dressing
Instructions:
Combine quinoa, tomatoes, cucumber, bell
pepper, red onion, feta, and olives in a bowl.
Drizzle with olive oil, lemon juice, and oregano
dressing.

Mediterranean Grilled Chicken Wrap:
Ingredients:
Grilled chicken breast, sliced
Whole grain wrap
Hummus
Tzatziki sauce
Sliced cucumber, tomatoes, and red onion
Fresh mint or parsley
Instructions:
Spread hummus on a whole grain wrap.
Layer with grilled chicken, tzatziki, sliced
cucumber, tomatoes, and red onion.
Garnish with fresh herbs and wrap.

Baked Falafel Bowl:
Ingredients:
Baked falafel patties
Quinoa or couscous, cooked
Mixed greens
Cherry tomatoes, halved
Cucumber, diced
Tahini dressing
Instructions:
Arrange baked falafel on a bed of quinoa or
couscous.
Add mixed greens, cherry tomatoes, and
cucumber.
Drizzle with tahini dressing.

Mediterranean Lentil Soup:
Ingredients:
Green or brown lentils
Carrots, celery, onion
Garlic, tomatoes
Spinach or kale
Olive oil, cumin, coriander, thyme

Instructions:
Sauté vegetables in olive oil until softened.
Add lentils, tomatoes, and spices; simmer until lentils are tender.
Stir in fresh greens before serving.

Grilled Eggplant and Halloumi Sandwich:
Ingredients:
Sliced eggplant, grilled
Halloumi cheese, grilled
Whole grain bread
Hummus
Tomato slices
Fresh basil leaves
Instructions:
Spread hummus on whole grain bread.
Layer with grilled eggplant, halloumi, tomato slices, and fresh basil.

5.3 **Dinner**

Mediterranean Grilled Salmon:
Ingredients:
Salmon filets
Lemon
Olive oil
Garlic, minced
Fresh dill
Cherry tomatoes, for garnish
Kalamata olives, sliced
Instructions:
Marinate salmon in a mixture of olive oil, lemon juice, minced garlic, and fresh dill.
Grill until salmon is cooked through.
Serve with a side of cherry tomatoes and sliced Kalamata olives.

Mediterranean Stuffed Bell Peppers:
Ingredients:
Bell peppers
Ground turkey or lean beef
Quinoa, cooked

Cherry tomatoes, diced
Feta cheese
Red onion, finely chopped
Garlic, minced
Olive oil, oregano, and thyme
Instructions:
Cut bell peppers in half and remove seeds.
Mix ground turkey or beef with cooked quinoa,
tomatoes, feta, red onion, garlic, and herbs.
Stuff peppers with the mixture and bake until
peppers are tender.

**Lemon-Herb Mediterranean Chicken
Skewers:**
Ingredients:
Chicken breast, cut into cubes
Lemon
Olive oil
Garlic, minced
Fresh rosemary and thyme
Cherry tomatoes, for skewering
Red onion, sliced

Instructions:
Marinate chicken in olive oil, lemon juice,
minced garlic, and fresh herbs.
Thread chicken, cherry tomatoes, and red
onion onto skewers.
Grill until chicken is cooked through.

**Mediterranean Shrimp and Vegetable
Stir-Fry:**
Ingredients:
Shrimp, peeled and deveined
Mixed vegetables (bell peppers, zucchini,
cherry tomatoes)
Garlic, minced
Olive oil
Lemon juice, oregano, and parsley
Whole wheat couscous or quinoa
Instructions:
Stir-fry shrimp and vegetables in olive oil and
minced garlic.
Season with lemon juice, oregano, and parsley.
Serve over cooked whole wheat couscous or
quinoa.

Mediterranean Ratatouille:
Ingredients:
Eggplant, zucchini, bell peppers, tomatoes
Onion, garlic
Olive oil, thyme, rosemary, oregano
Instructions:
Slice vegetables and layer in a baking dish.
Drizzle with olive oil and sprinkle with minced
garlic, thyme, rosemary, and oregano.
Bake until vegetables are tender.

Mediterranean Lentil and Vegetable Stew:
Ingredients:
Green or brown lentils
Carrots, celery, onion
Garlic, tomatoes
Spinach or kale
Olive oil, cumin, coriander, thyme
Instructions:
Sauté vegetables in olive oil until softened.
Add lentils, tomatoes, and spices; simmer until
lentils are tender.
Stir in fresh greens before serving.

5.4 **Snacks and Appetizers**

Hummus with Crudites:
Ingredients:
Hummus (chickpea dip)
Assorted raw vegetables (carrots, cucumber,
bell peppers)
Instructions:
Arrange a colorful assortment of raw
vegetables on a plate.
Serve with a bowl of hummus for dipping.

Greek Salad Skewers:
Ingredients:
Cherry tomatoes
Cucumber, diced
Feta cheese, cubed
Kalamata olives
Red onion, sliced
Instructions:
Thread cherry tomatoes, cucumber, feta,
olives, and red onion into small skewers.
Drizzle with olive oil and sprinkle with oregano.

Caprese Salad Bites:
Ingredients:
Cherry tomatoes
Fresh mozzarella cheese, cubed
Fresh basil leaves
Balsamic glaze
Instructions:
Skewer a cherry tomato, a cube of mozzarella,
and a fresh basil leaf on toothpicks.
Drizzle with balsamic glaze before serving.

Stuffed Grape Leaves (Dolma):
Ingredients:
Grape leaves (canned or fresh, blanched)
Rice
Pine nuts
Currants
Fresh dill and mint
Lemon juice

Instructions:
Mix cooked rice with pine nuts, currants, chopped dill, mint, and lemon juice.
Wrap the mixture in grape leaves and serve chilled.

Mediterranean Bruschetta:
Ingredients:
Whole grain baguette, sliced
Tomatoes, diced
Red onion, finely chopped
Kalamata olives, chopped
Feta cheese, crumbled
Fresh basil, chopped
Olive oil
Instructions:
Toast whole grain baguette slices.
Mix tomatoes, red onion, olives, feta, and basil.
Spoon the mixture onto the toasted bread and drizzle with olive oil.

Tzatziki with Pita Chips:
Ingredients:
Tzatziki sauce (Greek yogurt, cucumber, garlic, dill)
Whole wheat pita bread, cut into triangles
Instructions:
Prepare tzatziki by combining Greek yogurt, grated cucumber, minced garlic, and fresh dill. Serve with whole wheat pita chips for dipping.

Almonds and Figs:
Ingredients:
Raw almonds
Fresh or dried figs
Instructions:
Pair raw almonds with fresh or dried figs for a simple and satisfying snack.

Labneh topped with za'atar and olive oil:
Components:
strained yogurt, or labneh
Olive oil
Blend of spices called za'atar

Guidelines:
Transfer labneh onto a platter.
Add a za'atar sprinkle and drizzle with olive oil.

Roasted Red Pepper and Walnut Dip:
Ingredients:
Roasted red peppers
Walnuts
Garlic
Olive oil
Lemon juice
Instructions:
Blend roasted red peppers, walnuts, garlic,
olive oil, and lemon juice until smooth.
Serve with whole grain crackers or vegetable
sticks.

These snacks and appetizers embrace the
flavors of the Mediterranean diet, offering a mix
of textures, colors, and wholesome ingredients.
They're perfect for sharing or enjoying a light
and satisfying bite between meals.

CHAPTER SIX

6 Mediterranean Lifestyle

The Mediterranean lifestyle encompasses more than just a diet; it reflects the overall approach to living in the countries surrounding the Mediterranean Sea. This lifestyle has been associated with numerous health benefits, including lower rates of cardiovascular disease and longer life expectancy. Here's a comprehensive explanation of the Mediterranean lifestyle:

Mediterranean Diet:
Emphasis on Plant-Based Foods: The diet is rich in fruits, vegetables, whole grains, nuts, and legumes.
Healthy Fats: Olive oil is a primary source of fat, providing monounsaturated fats associated with heart health.

Moderate Protein: Lean protein sources such as fish, poultry, legumes, and limited red meat are preferred.

Dairy: Moderate consumption of dairy, with a focus on yogurt and cheese.

Wine in Moderation: Red wine, consumed in moderation during meals, is a common practice.

Physical Activity:

Regular Exercise: The Mediterranean lifestyle promotes regular physical activity, often in the form of walking, cycling, or engaging in outdoor activities.

Balanced Approach: Exercise is viewed as part of daily life, incorporating both structured activities and incidental movements.

Social Connections:

Emphasis on Socializing: The Mediterranean culture places importance on spending time with family and friends.

Shared Meals: Meals are often a communal affair, fostering social bonds and promoting a relaxed environment.

Mindful Eating:
Slow-Paced Meals: Meals are enjoyed at a leisurely pace, encouraging mindful eating and savoring the flavors.
Connection to Food: There's a strong connection to local and seasonal ingredients, with an appreciation for fresh, high-quality produce.

Relaxation and Stress Management:
Scheduled Breaks: Siestas, or afternoon naps, are common in some Mediterranean cultures, providing a break and promoting relaxation.
Outdoor Living: Enjoying nature and spending time outdoors contribute to stress reduction.

Cultural Practices:
Celebration of Festivals: Many
Mediterranean cultures celebrate festivals and
events with traditional foods, fostering a sense
of cultural identity.
Art and Creativity: An appreciation for art,
music, and cultural expression is integral to the
lifestyle.

Connection to Nature:
Proximity to the Sea: Many Mediterranean
communities have access to the sea, and a
connection to water is often associated with
relaxation and well-being.
Outdoor Activities: The region's climate
encourages outdoor activities like gardening,
hiking, and enjoying the natural surroundings.

Healthy Sleep Patterns:
Prioritizing Sleep: Adequate and quality sleep
is emphasized, contributing to overall
well-being and health.

Sustainable Practices:
Local and Seasonal Foods: The emphasis on local, seasonal produce supports sustainable and environmentally conscious practices.
Traditional Agricultural Methods: Some Mediterranean regions maintain traditional, sustainable farming practices.

Moderate Portions:
Balanced Meals: Meals are structured with a balance of macronutrients and are often composed of multiple smaller courses.
Portion Control: There is an emphasis on portion control, preventing overeating.

The Mediterranean lifestyle, encompassing diet, physical activity, social connections, and cultural practices, reflects a holistic approach to well-being. It emphasizes balance, enjoyment, and a connection to the surrounding environment, contributing to a healthier and more fulfilling life.

6.1 **Physical Activity**

Physical activity is an integral part of the Mediterranean lifestyle, complementing the health benefits derived from the Mediterranean diet. Here's an explanation of how physical activity is incorporated into the Mediterranean diet lifestyle:

Regular Exercise:
Outdoor Activities: The Mediterranean region's favorable climate often encourages outdoor activities, such as walking, cycling, hiking, and swimming.
Connection to Nature: The proximity to nature, including the sea and picturesque landscapes, provides an inviting environment for physical activities.

Daily Movement:
Incidental Exercise: Daily life in Mediterranean cultures often involves incidental movements, like walking to local markets, gardening, and other routine activities.

Work-Life Integration: Many Mediterranean communities integrate physical activity into daily life, such as walking to work or incorporating movement breaks during the day.

Social Exercise:
Group Activities: Social connections are valued, and group activities such as group walks, dancing, or playing sports are common.
Community Engagement: Community-based physical activities foster a sense of camaraderie and contribute to both physical and mental well-being.

Leisurely Pace:
Relaxed Approach: Exercise is not solely seen as a means to an end but is integrated into a more relaxed and enjoyable lifestyle.
Mindful Movements: Activities like yoga or tai chi, emphasizing mindfulness, are often practiced for their physical and mental benefits.

Celebration of Festivals and Events:
Traditional Dances: Festivals and events often involve traditional dances and physical activities, providing an opportunity for the community to come together in celebration.
Sports Events: Sporting events are common, ranging from local competitions to regional festivities.

Incorporation into Daily Routines:
Active Transportation: Walking or cycling is often used for transportation, integrating physical activity into daily commuting.
Agricultural Activities: In regions with agriculture, tending to crops and maintaining fields involve physical labor, contributing to daily activity levels.

Connection to the Sea:
Water-Based Activities: Proximity to the sea encourages water-based activities like swimming, sailing, or paddleboarding, providing a full-body workout.

Mind-Body Connection:
Yoga and Meditation: Practices that combine physical movement with mental well-being, such as yoga and meditation, are often embraced for a holistic approach to health.

Adaptation to Local Environment:
Mountainous Regions: In mountainous areas, activities like hiking and trekking are common.
Coastal Areas: Coastal regions may emphasize water sports and activities.

Lifestyle Integration:
Natural Integration: Physical activity is not treated as a separate or isolated component but is seamlessly integrated into the lifestyle, contributing to overall well-being.

The Mediterranean lifestyle recognizes the importance of staying active for health and vitality. Whether through structured exercises or daily movements integrated into life's routines, physical activity is woven into the fabric of the Mediterranean way of living. It aligns with the holistic approach to health, emphasizing not only a balanced diet but also an active and socially engaged lifestyle.

6.2 **Stress Management**

Stress management is a crucial aspect of the Mediterranean lifestyle, complementing the positive effects of the Mediterranean diet on overall well-being. Here's an explanation of how stress management is integrated into the Mediterranean diet lifestyle:

Emphasis on Relaxation:
Siesta Tradition: In some Mediterranean cultures, the tradition of taking a siesta (afternoon nap) is prevalent. This short break can contribute to stress reduction and improved alertness.

Outdoor Living:
Connection to Nature: The Mediterranean region's climate allows for ample outdoor living. Spending time outdoors, whether in gardens, parks, or near the sea, is associated with relaxation and stress relief.

Mediterranean Diet's Impact on Mood:
Nutrient-Rich Foods: The nutrient-dense foods in the Mediterranean diet, such as fruits, vegetables, and fatty fish, have been linked to improved mood and reduced risk of depression.
Omega-3 Fatty Acids: Fish, a staple in the Mediterranean diet, is rich in omega-3 fatty acids, which have been shown to have mood-stabilizing effects.

Shared Meals and Social Connections:
Communal Dining: Shared meals with family and friends provide an opportunity for social connections, fostering a sense of community and reducing feelings of isolation.
Communication and Support: Engaging in meaningful conversations during meals can contribute to emotional well-being and act as a form of stress relief.

Mindful Eating Practices:
Slow-Paced Meals: Meals in Mediterranean culture are often enjoyed at a leisurely pace, allowing individuals to savor flavors and practice mindful eating.
Focus on the Present Moment: Concentrating on the sensory experience of eating can help shift focus away from stressors.

Cultural Practices:
Cultural Celebrations: Engaging in cultural practices and celebrations can provide a break from daily stressors and add a sense of joy to life.
Festivals and Traditions: Participating in local festivals and traditions often involves music, dance, and communal activities that contribute to stress relief.

Physical Activity for Stress Reduction:
Regular Exercise: Physical activity, especially in the form of activities like walking, hiking, or yoga, is known to be effective in reducing stress and improving mood.

Adequate Sleep Patterns:
Prioritizing Sleep: The Mediterranean lifestyle values the importance of adequate and quality sleep, contributing to overall well-being and stress management.

Balanced Approach to Work and Life:
Work-Life Integration: The Mediterranean lifestyle often promotes a balanced approach to work and personal life, reducing the risk of burnout and chronic stress.

Mind-Body Techniques: Meditation and Yoga Mind-body therapies, like yoga and meditation, are popular because they help people cope with stress. These techniques can aid in fostering calmness of mind and relaxation.

6.3 **Social Connections**

Social connections play a significant role in the Mediterranean lifestyle, contributing to overall well-being and enhancing the positive effects of the Mediterranean diet. Here's an exploration of how social connections are emphasized in the Mediterranean lifestyle:

Family-Centric Culture:
Emphasis on Family: Mediterranean cultures often place a strong emphasis on family bonds and relationships.
Multigenerational Living: Many families live in close proximity or share households, fostering regular interaction and support.

Communal Dining:
Shared Meals: Meals are viewed as a time for family and friends to come together, share stories, and strengthen connections.

Extended Meal Times: The practice of leisurely, extended meals encourages meaningful conversations and enhances social connections.

Community Engagement:
Local Communities: Participation in local community activities, events, and festivals is common, fostering a sense of belonging.
Shared Celebrations: Celebrations often involve the community, reinforcing social bonds.

Outdoor Living and Socializing:
Public Spaces: Mediterranean communities often have vibrant public spaces, parks, and squares where people gather, promoting social interactions.
Outdoor Activities: The climate encourages outdoor activities, providing opportunities for neighbors and friends to engage in shared pursuits.

Cultural Practices:
Festivals and Traditions: Cultural events, festivals, and traditions bring people together, providing a shared sense of identity and connection.
Traditional Dances: Traditional dances and music are often enjoyed collectively.

Work-Life Balance:
Socializing at Work: The Mediterranean approach to work often involves socializing with colleagues, promoting camaraderie and a positive work environment.
Balanced Approach: A focus on work-life balance allows individuals to invest time in social relationships.

Intergenerational Interactions:
Respect for Elders: Respect for elders is a cultural norm, fostering strong intergenerational connections.

Wisdom Sharing: Elders play a crucial role in sharing wisdom, stories, and traditions with younger generations.

Local Markets and Shops:
Personal Connections: Shopping at local markets and small shops allows for personal connections with merchants and neighbors.
Community Support: Supporting local businesses creates a sense of community and interconnectedness.

Support Systems:
Community Support: In times of need, communities rally together to provide support, whether it's during celebrations or challenging circumstances.
Open-Door Policy: The idea of an open-door policy among neighbors is common, encouraging social interactions.

Physical Activities as Social Events:
Group Activities: Physical activities, such as group walks, sports, or dance classes, are often enjoyed in a social context.
Exercise as a Social Outlet: Regular exercise becomes a way to connect with others, contributing to both physical and mental well-being.

The emphasis on social connections in the Mediterranean lifestyle goes beyond mere socializing; it is deeply embedded in daily routines, cultural practices, and the way people approach relationships. This strong social fabric contributes to a sense of community, support, and shared joy, enhancing the overall quality of life.

CHAPTER SEVEN

7 Weekly Meal Plan

A Weekly Meal Plan for a Mediterranean diet cookbook typically emphasizes a balance of whole grains, fresh fruits and vegetables, lean proteins, and healthy fats. Here's a comprehensive example:

Day 1:
Breakfast: Greek yogurt with honey and mixed berries.
Lunch: Quinoa salad with cucumbers, cherry tomatoes, feta cheese, and olives.
Dinner: Grilled Mediterranean chicken with a side of roasted vegetables and couscous.

Day 2:
Breakfast: Oatmeal topped with sliced almonds and fresh peaches.
Lunch: Whole grain pita with hummus, falafel, and a Greek salad.
Dinner: Baked salmon with lemon and herbs, served with quinoa and steamed asparagus.

Day 3: Poached eggs and avocado slices served with whole grain bread for breakfast. Lunch consists of whole grain bread on the side and lentil soup.
Dinner is stuffed bell peppers in the Mediterranean manner with brown rice, ground turkey, tomatoes, and herbs.

Day 4:
Breakfast: Smoothie with spinach, banana, Greek yogurt, and a splash of olive oil.
Lunch: Whole wheat pasta with cherry tomatoes, garlic, olives, and grilled shrimp.
Dinner: Grilled eggplant and zucchini stack with tomato sauce and mozzarella.

Day 5:
Breakfast: Frittata with spinach, cherry tomatoes, and feta cheese.
Lunch: Chickpea salad with cherry tomatoes, red onions, and a lemon-tahini dressing.
Dinner: Herb-marinated grilled lamb chops with roasted sweet potatoes and green beans.

Day 6:
Breakfast: Whole grain pancakes with fresh strawberries and a drizzle of honey.
Lunch: Tuna and white bean salad with mixed greens and a balsamic vinaigrette.
Dinner: Mediterranean-style grilled swordfish with a side of quinoa and sautéed spinach.

Day 7:
Breakfast: Cottage cheese with sliced peaches and a sprinkle of chia seeds.
Lunch: Pita bread filled with grilled vegetables and topped with tzatziki sauce.

Dinner: Baked chicken breast with lemon, garlic, and rosemary, accompanied by roasted Brussels sprouts and bulgur.

Remember to adapt portion sizes based on individual needs and consult with a healthcare professional before making significant dietary changes.

7.1 Daily Breakfast, Lunch, Dinner, and Snack Ideas

Here is a detailed list of Mediterranean diet meal ideas for each day category:

Ideas for a Daily Breakfast:
Greek yogurt parfait topped with mixed berries, honey, and almonds.
tomato, feta cheese, spinach, and olives in an omelet.
Poached eggs and avocado slices served with whole grain toast.
spinach, banana, Greek yogurt, and a drizzle of olive oil combined into a smoothie.
Pancakes made with whole grains, garnished with a dollop of yogurt and fresh fruit.
Goat cheese, cherry tomatoes, and zucchini in a frittata.
Overnight oats with almond milk, chia seeds, and a selection of fruits.

Daily Lunch Ideas:

Quinoa salad with cucumber, cherry tomatoes, feta cheese, and olives.

Whole wheat pita with hummus, falafel, and a side of Greek salad.

Lentil soup with a whole grain roll.

Chickpea salad with cherry tomatoes, red onions, and a lemon-tahini dressing.

Tuna and white bean salad with mixed greens and balsamic vinaigrette.

Whole grain pasta with tomatoes, garlic, olives, and grilled shrimp.

Grilled vegetable and couscous bowl with a drizzle of tzatziki sauce.

Daily Dinner Ideas:

Grilled Mediterranean chicken with roasted vegetables and couscous.

Baked salmon with lemon and herbs, served with quinoa and asparagus.

Mediterranean-style stuffed bell peppers with ground turkey and brown rice.

Grilled eggplant and zucchini stack with tomato sauce and mozzarella.
Herb-marinated grilled lamb chops with sweet potatoes and green beans.
Swordfish grilled with Mediterranean spices, quinoa, and sautéed spinach.
Baked chicken breast with lemon, garlic, rosemary, Brussels sprouts, and bulgur.

Daily Snack Ideas:
Mixed nuts (almonds, walnuts, pistachios).
Fresh fruit slices with a small serving of cheese.
Hummus with carrot and cucumber sticks.
Greek yogurt with a sprinkle of granola.
Olives and cherry tomatoes.
Whole grain crackers with tzatziki.
Roasted chickpeas seasoned with Mediterranean spices.

CHAPTER EIGHT

8 Tips for Dining Out

When dining out on a Mediterranean diet, you can make mindful choices to align with the principles of this heart-healthy eating style. Here are some comprehensive tips:

Choose Olive Oil:
Opt for dishes that use olive oil as the primary source of fat. It's a staple in the Mediterranean diet and provides healthy monounsaturated fats.

Start with Vegetables:
Begin your meal with a salad or vegetable-based appetizer. This not only adds fiber and nutrients but also helps control your appetite.

Go for Seafood:
Mediterranean cuisine often features fish and
seafood. Choose grilled or baked options rich
in omega-3 fatty acids, such as salmon or
grilled shrimp.

Whole Grains:
Look for dishes that incorporate whole grains
like quinoa, bulgur, or whole wheat. This adds
fiber and additional nutrients to your meal.

Lean Proteins: Select lean protein sources
such as turkey, grilled chicken, or lentils. These
supply vital nutrients without having too many
saturated fats.

Embrace Herbs and Spices:
Mediterranean dishes are known for their
flavorful herbs and spices. Enjoy meals
seasoned with basil, oregano, garlic, and
rosemary instead of relying on salt.

Limit Processed Foods:
Minimize consumption of processed and fried foods. Stick to fresh, whole ingredients to get the most nutritional value.

Share Dishes:
Consider sharing appetizers or main courses to control portion sizes. This also allows you to taste a variety of dishes.

Ask for alterations: Don't hesitate to ask for alterations to suit your dietary preferences. To control the amount of sauces, ask for grilled instead of fried food or ask for them on the side.

Choose Legumes:
Opt for dishes that include beans, lentils, or chickpeas. These are rich in protein and fiber, contributing to the overall health benefits of the Mediterranean diet.

Enjoy Wine in Moderation:
If you enjoy alcohol, a glass of red wine can be
part of a Mediterranean-style meal. However,
moderation is key.

Eat mindfully by taking your time and enjoying
every meal. By practicing this skill, you can
avoid overeating by learning to recognize when
you're satisfied.

Hydrate with Water:
Drink water with your meal. It's a healthy
choice and helps maintain hydration.

Fruits for Dessert:
Opt for fresh fruits for dessert or share a
fruit-based option. It satisfies your sweet tooth
while staying in line with the diet.

Be Selective with Sweets:
If you choose a dessert, pick something that reflects Mediterranean ingredients, like a fruit sorbet or a small serving of baklava.

By incorporating these tips, you can make dining out an enjoyable and health-conscious experience while following the principles of the Mediterranean diet.

8.1 Making Healthy Choices at Restaurants

Scan the Menu Thoughtfully:
Look for dishes that feature vegetables, lean proteins, whole grains, and healthy fats like olive oil. Many Mediterranean-inspired options are labeled with terms like "grilled," "baked," or "roasted."

Start with a Salad:
Begin your meal with a fresh salad. Choose one with a variety of colorful vegetables, leafy greens, olives, and a drizzle of olive oil.

Choose Lean Proteins:
Opt for lean protein sources such as grilled chicken, fish, or legumes. These options align with the Mediterranean diet's emphasis on healthy proteins.

Emphasize Seafood:
Mediterranean cuisine often includes fish and seafood. Select grilled or baked fish dishes like salmon or trout for a boost of omega-3 fatty acids.

Customize Your Order:
Don't hesitate to customize your dish. Ask for grilled instead of fried, request sauces on the side, or inquire about whole grain options.

Select Whole Grains:
Look for dishes that incorporate whole grains like quinoa, bulgur, or brown rice. These choices provide fiber and essential nutrients.

Mind the Portions:
Pay attention to portion sizes. Consider sharing an entree or boxing up half of it to take home, especially if restaurant portions tend to be large.

Eat Less Processed Foods and Added Sugars: Steer clear of dishes that have a lot of processed ingredients or added sugars. Choose whole, fresh meals whenever you can.

Enjoy Vegetarian Options: Explore vegetarian options that include a variety of vegetables, legumes, and whole grains. Mediterranean cuisine offers many flavorful plant-based choices.

Herbs and Spices: Select recipes that call for herbs and spices such as rosemary, garlic, basil, and oregano. They enhance flavor without using an excessive amount of salt.

Mindful about Bread and Dips: If bread is served, choose whole grain options, and use them sparingly. Enjoy dips like hummus or tzatziki in moderation.

Hydrate with Water:
Opt for water or herbal tea instead of sugary beverages or excessive amounts of alcohol. Staying hydrated is a crucial part of a healthy dining experience.

Favor Healthy Fats:
Prioritize dishes that incorporate healthy fats like olive oil, nuts, and seeds. These contribute to the richness of flavors and align with the Mediterranean diet.

Be Discerning with Desserts:
Choose desserts that feature fruits or are smaller in portion size. Many Mediterranean desserts, like fruit sorbets or nut-based sweets, can be satisfying without excess sugar.

Listen to Your Body:
Pay attention to hunger and fullness cues. Eat slowly and enjoy your meal, stopping when you feel satisfied rather than overly full.

8.2 **FAQs and Troubleshooting**

The Mediterranean Diet: What Is It?
The customary eating habits of the nations that surround the Mediterranean Sea served as the model for the Mediterranean diet. It places a strong emphasis on whole grains, fruits, vegetables, legumes, nuts, and seeds. An important source of healthy fats is olive oil. It also limits red meat and processed meals and incorporates fish, chicken, and dairy in moderation.

Can I Follow the Mediterranean Diet if I'm Vegetarian or Vegan?
Yes, the Mediterranean Diet is adaptable to various dietary preferences. There are plenty of plant-based options such as fruits, vegetables, legumes, whole grains, and nuts. You can also incorporate plant-based proteins like tofu and tempeh.

How Can I Incorporate Olive Oil into My Cooking?

Use extra virgin olive oil for sautéing vegetables, drizzling over salads, and as a finishing touch to dishes. It adds a rich flavor and provides heart-healthy monounsaturated fats.

Are There Specific Portion Sizes I Should Follow?

The Mediterranean Diet doesn't strictly dictate portion sizes. However, it encourages moderation and balance. Listen to your body's hunger and fullness cues, and consider sharing larger dishes when dining out.

Can I Still Enjoy Desserts on the Mediterranean Diet?

Yes, but in moderation. Opt for desserts that incorporate fruits, nuts, or honey. Traditional Mediterranean sweets like baklava or fruit sorbets can be enjoyed occasionally.

Troubleshooting Tips:

**I Find It Challenging to Source
Mediterranean Ingredients. What
Can I Substitute?**
While authenticity is ideal, you can often find
substitutes for Mediterranean ingredients. For
instance, if a recipe calls for a specific type of
fish, consider using a locally available,
sustainable alternative.

**I'm Not a Fan of Certain Ingredients. Can I
Skip It?**
Absolutely. Mediterranean cuisine is flexible. If
you don't like a particular ingredient, feel free to
omit or substitute it with something you enjoy.
The goal is to make meals that suit your taste
preferences.

I'm Not Seeing the Expected Health Benefits. What Could be Wrong?

Health benefits may take time to manifest. Ensure you're incorporating a variety of fruits, vegetables, whole grains, and lean proteins. Also, consider factors like overall lifestyle, exercise, and stress management.

I'm Struggling to Find Time to Cook. Any Quick and Easy Recipes?

Look for recipes that require minimal preparation, such as one-pan dishes, salads, or quick stir-fries. Planning and prepping ingredients in advance can also save time during busy weekdays.

I'm Dining Out and It's Hard to Stick to the Diet. Any Tips?

Choose grilled or baked options, opt for salads, and ask for dressings or sauces on the side. Don't hesitate to customize your order to align with Mediterranean principles.

Remember, the Mediterranean Diet is about creating a sustainable and enjoyable way of eating. Feel free to adapt recipes to suit your preferences and lifestyle. If you have specific health concerns or questions, consulting a healthcare professional or dietitian is recommended.

8.2 Addressing Common Concerns

Concern: "Isn't Olive Oil High in Calories and Fat?"
Response: While olive oil is calorie-dense, it is a key component of the Mediterranean diet and a source of healthy monounsaturated fats. Moderation is crucial; use it for cooking and as a dressing in controlled amounts to benefit from its heart-healthy properties.

Concern: "I Don't Like Fish. Can I Still Follow the Mediterranean Diet?"
Response: Absolutely. While fish is a prominent protein source in the Mediterranean diet, it's not mandatory. You can focus on other lean proteins like poultry, legumes, and plant-based options such as tofu and tempeh.

Concern: "The Diet Seems Expensive with Special Ingredients. Is it Affordable?"
Response: The Mediterranean diet is based on whole, unprocessed foods, and many of its staples are affordable. Buy seasonal produce, grains, and legumes in bulk to save money. Focus on local alternatives if some ingredients are expensive or hard to find.

Concern: "I'm Not a Skilled Cook. Will the Recipes be Too Complicated?"
Response: The Mediterranean diet emphasizes simplicity. Many recipes involve basic cooking techniques like grilling, roasting, or sautéing. Start with easy recipes and gradually try more complex ones as you become more comfortable in the kitchen.

Concern: "I'm Concerned About Portion Sizes. How Can I Control Them?"
Response: Listen to your body's hunger and fullness cues.

Use smaller plates, share larger dishes when dining out, and be mindful of portion sizes. It's about balance and not feeling deprived.

Concern: "What if I Can't Find Mediterranean Ingredients Where I Live?"
Reaction: Adaptability is crucial, but authenticity is also valuable. Substitute local, similar ingredients for those that are hard to find. Fresh, whole foods are the foundation of the Mediterranean diet, so emphasize including them.

Concern: "I Have Dietary Restrictions. Can I Still Follow the Mediterranean Diet?"
Response: The Mediterranean diet is flexible and can be adapted to various dietary needs. If you have restrictions, such as gluten intolerance or lactose sensitivity, there are many alternative ingredients and recipes available.

"I'm not seeing weight loss," is the concern. How Should I Proceed?"

Reaction: Losing weight could take some time. Make sure you're handling stress and maintaining an active lifestyle in addition to the diet. Prioritize your general health over your weight loss. Seek guidance from a medical practitioner for specific recommendations.

Concern: "I'm Dining Out Frequently. How Can I Stick to the Diet?"

Response: Choose grilled or baked options, opt for salads, and customize your order to align with the Mediterranean diet. Be mindful of portion sizes and make choices that prioritize whole, fresh ingredients.

Concern: "I Have a Sweet Tooth. Can I Still Enjoy Desserts?"

Response: Absolutely. Choose desserts that feature fruits, nuts, or honey. Traditional Mediterranean sweets, when consumed in moderation, can be a delightful way to satisfy your sweet cravings.

8.3 Adapting the Diet to Individual Needs

The Mediterranean diet is known for its flexibility, making it adaptable to various preferences, dietary restrictions, and individual needs. Here's how you can customize the diet to suit your unique requirements:

Personal Preferences:
Approach: Embrace the diversity within the Mediterranean diet. If you have preferences for certain ingredients or flavors, focus on incorporating those while staying true to the overall principles of the diet.

Vegetarian or Vegan Lifestyle:
Approach: The Mediterranean diet is easily adaptable for vegetarians and vegans.

Increase your consumption of plant-based proteins like legumes, tofu, and tempeh. Utilize a variety of colorful vegetables, fruits, nuts, and whole grains.

Gluten-Free Needs:

Approach: Substitute gluten-containing grains like wheat with gluten-free alternatives such as quinoa, brown rice, or gluten-free pasta. Pay attention to labels and choose naturally gluten-free foods like fruits, vegetables, and lean proteins.

Lactose Intolerance:

Approach: Opt for lactose-free or low-lactose dairy options if you still want to include dairy in your diet. Alternatively, explore plant-based milk alternatives such as almond, soy, or oat milk.

Nut Allergies:

Approach: Replace nuts with seeds like sunflower seeds, pumpkin seeds, or chia seeds for a similar nutritional boost. Ensure that recipes are adjusted to exclude nuts or use safe alternatives.

Seafood Preferences:

Approach: If you don't enjoy or cannot consume seafood, focus on other lean protein sources such as poultry, legumes, eggs, or plant-based proteins. Make sure to incorporate a variety of these alternatives for a balanced diet.

Limited Cooking Skills or Time

Constraints:

Approach: Start with simple recipes that require minimal cooking skills. Look for quick and easy options like salads, one-pan dishes, or grilled proteins with a side of vegetables. As you gain confidence, you can explore more complex recipes.

Medical Conditions (e.g., Diabetes, Hypertension):
Approach: Consult with a healthcare professional or a registered dietitian to tailor the Mediterranean diet to your specific health needs. They can provide guidance on managing conditions through appropriate food choices and portion control.

Weight Loss Goals:
Approach: While the Mediterranean diet is associated with various health benefits, including weight management, individual responses may vary. Focus on portion control, listen to your body's hunger cues, and incorporate regular physical activity.

Cultural or Religious Dietary Restrictions:
Approach: Modify recipes to align with cultural or religious dietary restrictions. Replace ingredients as needed while still emphasizing the core principles of the Mediterranean diet.

Athletes or Active Individuals:
Approach: Adjust portion sizes to meet increased energy needs. Ensure an adequate intake of protein, whole grains, and healthy fats to support energy levels and recovery.

Picky Eaters or Children:
Approach: Involve picky eaters in meal planning and preparation. Experiment with various flavors and textures, and gradually introduce them to new Mediterranean ingredients. Offer choices to accommodate preferences.

Remember, the key to successfully adapting the Mediterranean diet is finding a balance that suits your lifestyle, preferences, and health goals. It's a flexible and inclusive approach that encourages creativity and enjoyment of a wide variety of nutritious foods. If you have specific concerns or questions, seek guidance from healthcare professionals or nutrition experts.

CONCLUSION

Embarking on a journey with the Mediterranean Diet Cookbook for beginners offers not just a collection of recipes but a holistic approach to embracing a lifestyle rooted in health, flavor, and cultural richness. Throughout this culinary exploration, we've delved into the core principles of the Mediterranean diet, providing a comprehensive guide for those taking their first steps on this nutritious path.

The beauty of the Mediterranean diet lies in its adaptability, making it accessible for individuals with various dietary needs, preferences, and lifestyles. Whether you're a vegetarian, dealing with food allergies, or navigating a busy schedule, the recipes and tips provided empower you to tailor this eating style to suit your individual requirements.

From substituting ingredients to adjusting portion sizes, the Mediterranean diet encourages a personalized approach that promotes sustainable, enjoyable eating habits.

Our journey through daily meal plans, dining-out tips, and troubleshooting common concerns has underscored the versatility of this culinary tradition. We've discovered how to navigate restaurant menus, make mindful choices, and address potential challenges, ensuring that the benefits of the Mediterranean diet can be seamlessly incorporated into diverse lifestyles.

In essence, the Mediterranean Diet Cookbook for beginners serves as a gateway to a world of delicious, nourishing meals that prioritize whole foods, lean proteins, and heart-healthy fats.

By embracing the use of olive oil, an array of fresh fruits and vegetables, and the vibrant flavors of herbs and spices, individuals can cultivate a sustainable and satisfying relationship with food.

As you embark on this culinary adventure, remember that the Mediterranean diet isn't just about the recipes—it's about cultivating a lifestyle that celebrates health, joy, and longevity. Whether you're savoring a colorful Greek salad, indulging in a plate of grilled fish, or enjoying a simple fruit parfait, each meal is an opportunity to nourish both body and soul.

In conclusion, the Mediterranean Diet Cookbook for beginners serves as a compass, guiding you toward a lifestyle that seamlessly integrates healthful eating into your daily routine. Embrace the rich tapestry of flavors, experiment with diverse ingredients, and savor the joy of creating meals that not only contribute to your well-being but also connect you to the vibrant culinary traditions of the Mediterranean. Cheers to a journey of culinary discovery and a life well-lived through the nourishing embrace of the Mediterranean diet.

Thank you for embarking on this flavorful journey with the Mediterranean Diet Cookbook for beginners. We hope these recipes have inspired you to embrace a lifestyle filled with delicious, nutritious, and culturally rich meals.

As you savor the vibrant flavors and nourishing ingredients, remember that each dish is a step towards a healthier and more joyful you. The Mediterranean diet isn't just about what you eat; it's a celebration of life, well-being, and the joy of sharing delicious moments with loved ones.

We appreciate your time and commitment to exploring this culinary adventure. May your kitchen continue to be a place of creativity, health, and happiness. Here's to a future filled with tasty discoveries and a lifetime of good eating!